Jen
50.
Rig
Left on Hyattsville

This journal belongs to

____